Herbal Magic:

Wicca Beginner guide to Herbs and plants for Rituals and Spells

Scott Markson

© Copyright 2018 by Scott Markson- All rights reserved.

The following book is reproduced below with the goal of providing information that is as accurate and as reliable as possible. Regardless, purchasing this book be consent to the fact that both the publisher and the author of this book are in no way experts on the topics discussed within, and that any recommendations or suggestions made herein are for entertainment purposes only. Professionals should be consulted as needed before undertaking any of the action endorsed herein.

This declaration is deemed fair and valid by both the American Bar Association and the Committee of Publishers Association and is legally binding throughout the United States.

Furthermore, the transmission, duplication or reproduction of any of the following work, including precise information, will be considered an illegal act, irrespective of whether it is done electronically or in print. The legality extends to creating a secondary or tertiary copy of the work or a recorded copy and is only allowed with an expressed written consent of the Publisher. All additional rights are reserved.

The information in the following pages is broadly considered to be a truthful and accurate account of facts, and as such any inattention, use or misuse of the information in question by the reader will render any resulting actions solely under their purview. There are no scenarios in which the publisher or the original author of this work can be in any fashion deemed liable for any hardship or damages that may befall them after undertaking information described herein.

Additionally, the information found on the following pages is intended for informational purposes only and should thus be considered, universal. As befitting its nature, the information presented is without assurance regarding its continued validity or interim quality. Trademarks that mentioned are done without written consent and can in no way be considered an endorsement from the trademark holder.

Your Free Gift

As a way of saying thank you for your purchase, I wanted to offer you a free bonus e-book called **My Little Book Of Wicca Spells**

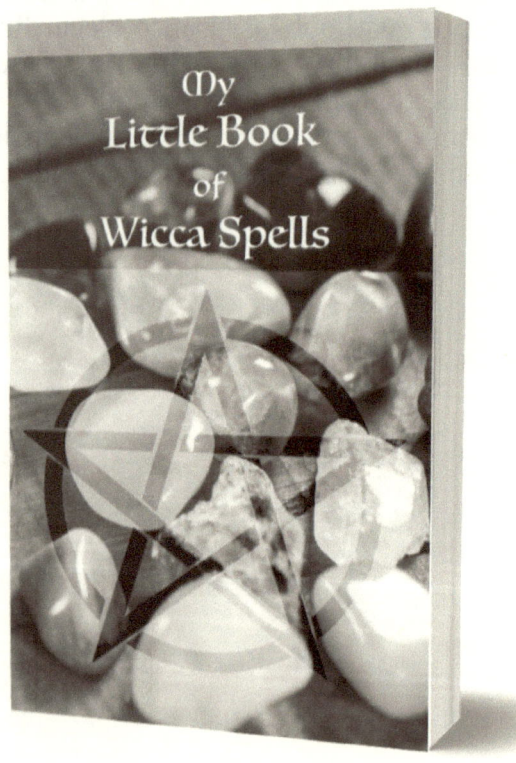

Download the free ebook here:
https://www.subscribepage.com/wiccaspells

Spells can have a powerful effect on yourself and the surrounds around you. This free ebook has 9 invigorating spells that can help protect your home, bring about luck and help in your careers.

Listen to this book for free

Do you want to be able to listen to this book whenever you want? Maybe whilst driving to work or running errands. It can be difficult nowadays to sit down and listen to a book. So I am really excited to let you know that this book is available in audio format. What's great is you can get this book for FREE as part of a 30-day audible trial. Thereafter if you don't want to stay an Audible member you can cancel, but keep the book.

Benefits of signing up to audible:
- After the trial, you get 1 free audiobook and 2 free audio originals each month
- Can roll over any unused credits
- Choose from over 425,000 + titles
- Listen anywhere with the Audible app and across multiple devices
- Keep your audiobooks forever, even if you cancel your membership

Click below to get started
Audible US - https://tinyurl.com/yxrp9dbg
Audible UK - https://tinyurl.com/y3vxbaa4
Audible FR - https://tinyurl.com/y2oqpl9q
Audible DE - https://tinyurl.com/y4udansp

Table of Contents

INTRODUCTION 1
CHAPTER 1: WICCA BASICS 3

   THE WICCAN REDE AND RULE OF THREE 4
   THE TRADITIONAL TOOLS OF WICCA 6
   PURIFYING THE RITUAL SPACE 9
   SIMPLE CONSECRATION RITUAL FOR TOOLS 12
   THE RITUAL 13

CHAPTER 2: THE USE OF HERBS AND PLANTS IN WICCA 17

   TOOLS FOR HERBAL PREPARATIONS 20
   DIFFERENT HERBAL PREPARATIONS USED IN WICCA 23
      Drying Herbs 23
      Water-Based Herbal Mixtures 24
      Oil-Based Herbal Mixtures 25
      Alcohol-Based Herbal Mixtures 27

CHAPTER 3: ENCYCLOPEDIA OF IMPORTANT HERBS EVERY WITCH SHOULD UNDERSTAND 29

CHAPTER 4: AN HERBAL BOOK OF SHADOWS 43

   HERBAL LOVE SPELLS 45
      Honey Jar Attraction Spell 45
      Herbal Love Perfume 47
      Spell for Burning Desire 49
   HERBAL WEALTH & LUCK SPELLS 51
      Chalice of Plenty 51
      Money Sachet Spell 53
      The Money Orange 55
      Luck Pouch 57
      Good Luck Bath 58
   HERBAL PROTECTION & HEALTH SPELLS 60
      Home Protection Spell 60
      Witch Jar 62
      Positivity Magnet Spell 64
      Healing Power of Three Spell 66
      Beauty Bath 68
      Herbal Dream and Sleep Spells 69
      Herbal Dream Sachet 69
      Herbal Sleeping Sachet Spell 71

CHAPTER 5: WHERE TO BUY AND HOW TO GROW & FORAGE HERBS FOR MAGICAL USAGE....................... 73

- Buying Herbs 74
- Growing Herbs 77
- Foraging for Herbs 78

CHAPTER 6: FURTHER RESOURCES 81

- Books on Wicca and Magic: 81
- Books on Foraging for Plants: 83
- Resources for Growing Plants 85

CONCLUSION 87

Introduction

Congratulations on downloading *Herbal Magic: Wicca Beginner guide to Herbs and plants for Rituals and Spells.*

Wicca has fascinated people for generations and there are countless books about it, but most of them are written by expert witches, for other expert witches to read. This book takes on a more introductory tone and focuses that introduction on a single aspect of Wicca: the use of herbs and plants in Wicca magic.

Herbs and plants have been used in magical practice since before recorded history, and they play a vital role in the modern practice of Wicca. This book will explore how herbs and plants are used by modern witches, including the different types of herbal preparations. It also includes several herbal-based spells with easy to follow instructions so the reader can put theory into practice.

Further chapters provide a brief encyclopedia detailing several of the most important herbs, some of their most common uses, the best places to source herbs for magical uses, as well as tips on growing or foraging herbs.

There are plenty of books on this subject on the market, thanks again for choosing this one! Every effort was made to ensure it is full of as much useful information as possible, please enjoy!

Chapter 1: Wicca Basics

Wicca can be a difficult concept to introduce to newcomers because it encompasses such a diverse practice, with thousands of different groups and individuals using the term to describe their unique beliefs and rituals. Instead of focusing on a single Wiccan tradition or belief system, this book will take a more general path. The use of herbs in Wiccan magic transcends the different traditions. One can use the information provided in this book, whether they are the strictest Gardnerian Wiccan or a chaos magic practicing neo-pagan.

This chapter will provide an overview of the fundamental beliefs held in common by most Wicca. This will include a description of the traditional tools used in the practice of Wicca as well as provide a simplified version of the Wiccan Ritual. For those new to Wicca, this will provide a starting point that can be used as is, or incorporated into their own practice as they see fit. Outside of a few fundamental concepts, there are few hard and fast rules in the practice of Wicca.

As a religious belief, Wicca is generally duotheistic, believing in two gods, the male and female, the God and Goddess. Being such a diverse group, some practitioners view them under a more pantheistic light. To them, the God and Goddess are evident in everything in the natural world. Others beliefs tend towards polytheism, believing in pantheons of Gods and Goddesses, often existing panthea such as those worshipped by the ancient Greeks or Norse. Still, others view the idea of the God and Goddess as concepts and not actual beings. It can be easy to see why Wicca is such a difficult concept to introduce when it can be so diverse.

The Wiccan Rede and Rule of Three

Regardless of their beliefs on the divine, Wiccans have a fundamental respect for nature and a desire to live in harmony with both others and the natural world itself. This idea forms the basis for Wicca's two foundational beliefs: The Wiccan Rede and the Rule of Three. Again, with such great diversity, almost every Wiccan tradition has their own wording for these rules, which might differ from the version used in the book but underneath, the meaning is generally the same.

The Wiccan Rede is the Wiccan version of the Golden Rule: as long as it harms none, do what thou wilt. A simple reading of this is that a Wiccan Practitioner is free to do whatever they want, including their use of magic, for any purpose as long as nobody else is harmed. This prohibits the use of spells to harm others, both emotionally and physically, as well as any actions that will cause others harm. This is the backbone for Wiccan morality though it has a practical aspect that will be shown in the Rule of Three.

Interpreting the Rede at a deeper level, however, illuminates another side to it. The word 'wilt' in the Rede is an older version of the word 'will' and most view its use in the Rede to mean as one desires or wants but can also refer to willpower. "Do what thou wilt" in that context, refers to doing what your own willpower or volition desires. This can be a subtle distinction but the concept behind it is meant to add a layer of self-reflection, to question whether one's actions and desires are truly what one wills.

An example is the easiest way to show this distinction—let us start with a Wiccan who is addicted to cocaine. To start with, there are multiple ways her actions here could harm others. The illegal trade of 'drug traffic' is more in human misery all throughout the supply chain, so purchasing those drugs contributes to the harming of others. One's actions, while on these drugs, can result in harm and they can cause issues with the consumer themselves. Harming oneself often harms those who love the person. Moving to will, feeding an addiction can be what a person desires or wants to do, but it isn't really their own volition. They are being led by their desires, instead of leading and determining their own actions. "Do what thou wilt" isn't really carte blanche to do anything at all.

As the Wiccan Rede is the Wiccan golden rule, the Rule of Three is the foundation of Wiccan metaphysical beliefs when it comes to the practice of magic. Again, the wording will differ between Wiccan traditions, but at its basic, the Rule of Three states that whatever energy they put out into the world, may it be good or bad, returns to them threefold. This relates to the type of magical energy used in their spells and is similar to the Dharmic definition of karma. Generally, performing spells that have an underlying positive intent—a luck spell before a job interview— will return positive energy to the caster, while casting spells with negative intent—a curse on another candidate for the same job—will manifest a negative energy to the caster.

As with almost anything Wicca related, there are groups that follow radically different versions of the Rede and Rule of Three. In the end, what to follow is up to the practitioner and what their beliefs and experiences will shape. The Rede and Rule of Three presented here can be seen as guides, hard and fast rules, or they can be discounted completely, though the latter likely comes with unforeseen consequences.

The Traditional Tools of Wicca

The center of the Wiccan religious belief and traditional magic is the *Ritual*. This can consist akin to the religious services common in other religions. Just like those other religions, the ritual in Wicca often requires the use of ritual tools. Wicca has four tools used in the Wiccan ritual, and each of these tools is associated with one of the four elements. These tools are the **Athame** representing fire, the **Chalice** representing water, the **Pentacle** representing earth, and the **_Wand_** representing air.

A more traditional practitioner of Wicca will often have specially made versions of these tools that are only used in their ritual room, for ritual purposes only; less traditional practitioners might improvise their tools. Regardless of the reverence, the practitioner holds for their tools, almost all will consecrate their tools before use. A simple consecration ritual is provided in the next section along with a basic ritual.

An **_Athame_** is a ritual dagger, and out of all the traditional tools, it is the most used. It is the focus of magical energies that the practitioner directs and is used to carve symbols into the candle, as well as in drawing the Circle. A double-edged dagger is the most common among traditional practitioners, and it is often decorated with symbols of importance to its owner. Nontraditionalists can use any bladed tool as an _Athame_ though they should wash and consecrate it first. A word of warning here, while washing and consecrating the blade should remove any negative energy and make the blade suitable for magical uses, blades can house a multitude of negative energy that can accumulate over time. Even a blade that accidentally cut a person can keep those negative energies until they fester. A blade that was used intentionally to cause harm to another can have even more negative energies attached. If using a blade with an unknown origin, cleansing it of any negative energy is a good idea.

The **Pentacle** is generally a disk that is inscribed with a *pentagram* that is surrounded by a circle. This represents the four elements, as well as the divine or spirit as the fifth element. *Pentacles* of various materials are available, although most practitioners prefer one made of natural materials such as wood, stone or even metal, instead of plastics. Nontraditionalists often improvise their *pentacles*, painting or drawing a *pentacle* on a nice piece of paper makes an easy pentacle for the practitioner on a budget. In the ritual, *pentacles* are generally the centerpiece and placed on the altar where they are used to charge or consecrate other tools or items used in spells.

The **Wand** will be familiar to most people based on its use by fantasy magicians like in the *Harry Potter* books. However, Wiccan *wands* can be made of any material, though as with pentacles, natural materials are preferred over plastics. For the practitioner on a budget, a found stick can easily become a *wand* as can a cut branch. These can become powerful objects with a personal meaning for the practitioner. Cutting a branch from a tree that has personal meaning, for use as a *wand* is often best, and the practitioner can further personalize it with symbols important to them. In practice, a *wand* can be used in place of the *Athame* for most uses outside carving and is often preferred in spells where the use of a weapon could be counterproductive to the purpose of the spell.

A *silver goblet* is the traditional version of the **Chalice,** though any container that can contain water will suffice as a *chalice,* as long as it is properly cleaned and consecrated. Silver is common because of its connection to the Moon and thus the Goddess, but any natural product can be used, including glass. The *chalice* generally holds consecrated water or wine in a ritual, as well as other liquids when they are required for a specific spell. It is often passed around the group or coven when performing a ritual with other people.

In addition to the common tools, the Ritual requires an **Altar** as the centerpiece of the ritual space. This can be as simple as a small table that can hold the tools used in the ritual, or it can be specifically built for ritual use. In the end, any flat surface can act as an *altar*. Additional tools that are used in most spells are *candles* and *incense*—which are quite common. *Crystals* are used by some practitioners as well, and a multitude of *herbs* and *oils* can be used in both the ritual and spells.

Purifying the Ritual Space

Rituals are generally performed in a ritual space. This can be a special room used only for rituals and spells but more often, it is a room such as a den or dining room that is used for other purposes as well. Outdoor rituals are also common, especially on important holidays such as equinoxes and during the full moon. Before ritual use, the ritual space needs to be purified. The first step in this is just general cleaning, though while tidying the ritual space, many practitioners focus on the intent of the ritual to strengthen the positive energies in the ritual space.

When the ritual space is physically clean, the purifying ritual can start. This requires an altar with four items arranged at the cardinal compass points. A small dish of salt is set to the north, representing earth. Next to that, to the east, is incense representing air. For this ritual, stick incense is best, as it will be lit by a candle. The choice of incense is up to the practitioner and most would pick one based on the spells they intend to cast, or one used for purification such as a smudge stick.

A container of water is set to the west. At this stage, do not use your ritual chalice, as you will be purifying it in the next ritual. It is important that this container can easily be carried because it will be moved around the ritual space. Finally, to the south, set a candle to represent fire. An additional candle is placed in the center of the altar and lit before the ritual starts. The colors of candles can be important for some rituals. For purification, white is the standard choice, but it really is up to the practitioner and using candles of specific colors can work better in different rituals.

If possible, five additional candles are placed on the outskirts of the ritual space. To place these candles, imagine a large pentagram on the floor of the ritual space and place the candles at the points of the pentagram. They are unlit at the begging of the purifying ritual.

Practitioners often speak during rituals, invoking the spirits or the goddess to bless the ritual space, as well as granting power to the spells they are casting. Given the huge amount of different beliefs within Wicca, this chapter omits the spoken word from the rituals, so that the reader can add their own based on their specific beliefs.

Light the central candle and turn off any electronic lights in the room before returning to the altar. Hold your right hand over the dish of salt and envision the powers of the earth granting their strength to purify and consecrate the ritual space. Take a pinch of salt in your right hand and move it over to the container of water. Sprinkle the salt in the water, envisioning the cleansing power of the spirits of the water as well as its life-giving nature.

Pick up the container of water and swirl it with your finger envisioning it filling with cleansing and purifying power. Walk around the ritual room and flick the salt water to purify the space, envisioning the purifying power in the salt water with every flick. There is no set rule for how many times this is performed, but at the very least, a flick at each of the five points of the pentagram is used; anyone else performing the ritual should dip their finger in the container and flick themselves for ritual purification.

Return to the altar and take the central candle in your right hand. Move it to the candle placed to the south and light the candle, envisioning the cleansing power of fire. Next, move the candle to the incense, lighting it while envisioning the spirits of the air blessing and purifying the space.

Take the incense in your right hand and walk around the ritual space, pausing at each of the points of the pentagram as well as in front of any other people present to ritually purify them. Return to the altar and place the incense back into position. The ritual space is now ritually clean. You can proceed with cleansing the ritual tools, and then the ritual—or you can perform the ritual cleansing well before the actual ritual.

Simple Consecration Ritual for Tools

Before using any tool in a ritual or spell, it is important to clean and consecrate them. This step removes any negative or even just unfocused energy from the items. The reason this is important is that those energies can mingle and change the energies used in performing the ritual or spell, increasing the chance of failure, or contaminating the intent of the spell, twisting its effects into something the caster did not desire.

The consecration ritual for the tools is an extension of the purification ritual for the ritual space. Once the space has been purified, return to the altar with the tools that need to be purified. One at a time, take the tools and anoint them first with the salt water, envisioning the cleansing power removing any negative energies from the tool. The amount of time taken here will depend on the possible negative energies in the tool. If it is the first time you have used a particular tool, especially if you do not know its history, you might need to cleanse it longer than a tool that is regularly used in rituals. Use your intuition to feel for the energies of an item.

Next, pass the tool over the flame of the candle while envisioning the cleaning power of fire. Flammable items should be held higher above the flame. The purpose is to ritually cleanse the item, not to burn it! Finally, pass the tool over the incense, envisioning the powers of the spirits of the air blessing and cleansing the tool. Once you have finished doing this with the tools that you intend to use in the ritual, you can remove the cleansing items from the altar, and get ready for the actual ritual.

The Ritual

The Ritual starts with the casting of the circle, which serves a dual purpose. The circle protects the ritual space and its occupants from any outside energies that could infect the ritual or spell. This protection also serves to concentrate the energies created within the circle by keeping them inside the circle for the duration of the ritual or spell casting. Generally, once the circle has been cast, the practitioner and anyone else involved in the ritual should be within it for the duration of the spell or the ritual.

Casting the circle starts with lighting the candles. Take the central candle from the altar and approach the candle at the top of the imaginary pentagram in the ritual room. Light that candle, and then move counter-clockwise to light the other four candles. Once you reach the top of the pentagram, return the central candle to the altar. Now, take the Athame in your right hand and approach the top candle again. Hold out your arm with the Athame over the candle for a moment and walk around the room counter-clockwise, holding the Athame over each of the other candles. Once you have reached the top candle again, the circle has been cast.

With the circle cast, the next step is to draw down the divine. The intention here is to invite the divine power into the circle to imbue it and the people inside it with the divine power. Take your Athame or wand in your right hand and hold it to the sky. Stare up and envision the power of the divine entering the Athame or wand, charging it with power and energy. Hold this position until you feel the power, and then move the tip of the Athame or wand to your heart, envisioning the divine power entering your body and flowing to the tips of your toes and the top of your head.

The next part of the ritual is the casting of spells. Multiple spells can be cast and if the ritual is performed by more than one person, others can have a chance to cast their own spells, drawing down the divine, for each new spell or caster.

With the spells cast, there is only one more section of the ritual: Communion, commonly called *'cakes and ale'* by most Wiccan groups. This is generally only done when performing a ritual with others. Any beverage can be used, but wine or beer is the most common. As for the cakes, any homemade cookie or pastry will suffice.

Return to the altar and pour the wine into the chalice, envisioning the powers of the earth that provided a home for the vine and the water that fed it. Think on how the grape became the wine and how it provides sustenance to you. Take a sip and then move to the other participants and offer the chalice to them.

Back at the altar, place the cookies on the pentacle and envision the seeds sprouting from the earth and the water feeding the plants. Think on how the plant became grain and then flour to provide substance to you. Take a cookie and then offer one to all the other participants. Return the pentacle to the altar and then enjoy the company of the other participants for as long as desired.

To open the circle and end the ritual, return to the altar and take your Athame into your right hand. Point it to the north, and thank the spirits of the earth for their presence in the circle during the ritual; turn to the west, and thank the spirits of the water for their presence in the circle; turn to the south, and thank the powers of fire and finally, facing to the east, thank the powers of the air. Hold your Athame to the sky and envision the powers of the divine that you called into the circle returning to their source. The circle has opened and the ritual is complete.

This is just one example of a ritual and it is a simple version of the traditional ritual. What will work for you could be different. Shorter rituals for spell work can work for some, while others prefer the more traditional rituals. There is no wrong way to do it and the more experience you have, the better you will be at tailoring the ritual to your needs.

Chapter 2: The Use of Herbs and Plants in Wicca

The use of plants in magic is an ancient tradition that likely predates the written word. Our Neolithic ancestors foraged the forests and found plants and mushrooms that, when eaten, would grant them an altered state of consciousness. These magical plants and the visions they caused became central to the spiritual life of our prehistoric ancestors, and their use as spiritual aids continues to this day in certain groups.

In addition to any psychoactive plants found and used by these Neolithic hunter-gatherers, they discovered that certain plants could provide health benefits. Adding a certain flower to drinking water might soothe a sore throat, chewing on the leaves of a different plant might take the pain of a headache away. This became the basis for traditional or folk medicine, used for thousands of generations.

For the early shamans and magicians, these healing herbs—as well as other plants—became important tools for their magic and ritual. Over time, they refined this knowledge through experimentation and spell work, learning which plants provided the most magical energies to certain types of magic. A tradition of herbal magic came into being everywhere people lived, using the local plants, with knowledge passed down through the ages, known for their particular powers and proclivities.

The modern practitioner of the Wiccan arts is in a much luckier position. Generations of shamans, wise women of the woods, alchemist, and magicians have passed their knowledge of the magical properties of herbs and other plants, down the generations. This saves the modern practitioner the need for experimentation, though most perform a few, as they become more familiar with certain spells and herbs to discover the most powerful combinations.

The ease of global trade provides the modern practitioner another benefit the ancient shamans lacked: the ability to obtain the plants needed for their magic even if they only grow on the other side of the planet. Our ancestral shamans had to make do with the plants they could gather on their own from their immediate environment. If they were lucky, they might have some access to a rudimentary trade network that could provide some plants that grew elsewhere, but that shaman's knowledge would be limited to what they were taught, limited to the plants their mentor used. They would have little knowledge of how to use new plants.

Today, anyone living near a moderately stocked grocery store has access to a multitude of edible herbs from a garden center and maybe a flower shop as well, as they have access to a lot more.

With an internet connection, they can get almost any plant, save those that have been deemed illegal to own. The generations of recorded knowledge pertaining to the powers of different plants are also easily available to the modern practitioner, enabling them to quickly learn the best way to use the herbs their ancestors would have never seen.

The final benefit the modern practitioner has over the ancient shamans is the multitude of ways they can use herbs and other plants in their magic. Those ancient shamans likely had access to fire, maybe even a rudimentary clay kiln to produce clay vessels for the boiling of water. Today, in addition to fire and water, the modern practitioner has distilled alcohol, sugar, refined oils, and other tools that can be used for the preparation of herbs and other plants to be used in their magic.

This chapter will provide an overview of several different methods that the modern practitioner of Wicca prepare, like herbs and other plants for different magical purposes. It will also contain a description of some of the different tools used in the preparation of herbs. The following chapters will detail the several different important herbs and plants used in herbal magic, as well as providing several basic spells for their use and a guide to buying, foraging, and growing your own herbs.

Tools for Herbal Preparations

Many of the herbs used in magic are also used as food, so many of the herbs for magical uses will already be available in a stocked kitchen and can be used for both purposes. Many practitioners prefer to have a separate version of these tools that are used specifically for magic. There are three benefits to this. First, as the other tools used in Wicca, it is best to purify and cleanse them of any negative powers or energies. While this isn't a critique of anybody's cooking skills, negative energies can build up from using a vessel for cooking between the preparations of the herbs for magical purposes. Having dedicated tools for magic require less purification, as they wouldn't build up negative energy between magical preparations.

Another benefit of having a separate set of tools for magical purposes is safety. While most of the herbs and plants used in magic can be safely consumed, there are a few that can cause digestive issues or are even toxic to humans. Preparing any of these herbs with tools that are also used in food preparation can lead to cross-contamination. The final benefit is in the transference of energies from your dedicated magical tools to the herbal preparations. One can chop herbs for a spell with any knife, but using the Athame they had been using in their rituals for years will boost the potency of the spell and attune it better to their own energies.

Tools that most practitioners would likely find helpful in addition to their standard kitchen tools such as pots, pans, knives, and cutting boards, are a mortar & pestle, strainers or cheesecloth, funnels, as well as large canning jars and dark glass bottles for storage. Light is often the enemy when it comes to different herbal concoctions, just like wine, which makes clean wine bottles ideal for the storage of herbal liquids. The funnels and strainers are used to remove solids from herbal liquids and to move them into bottles.

The mortar & pestle is a grinding tool used since prehistory. It consists of a bowl— the mortar— usually made out of ceramic or carved from a hard stone, though hardwoods and metal are also sometimes used. The Pestle is a heavy club-shaped stick usually made from the same material as the Mortar. To use, a person places the ingredients to be ground in the mortar and then presses the pestle head into the mortar bowl and rotate it until it is pulverized to the desired level. They are commonly used in food preparations for both grinding spices as well as wet mixtures. Pesto, for example, gets its name for its preparation using a mortar and pestle. They were also traditionally used by pharmacists to grind ingredients to make medicines.

For magical uses, most practitioners favor a stone mortar & pestle. Stone is heavy and strong, allowing for better grinding. It is also relatively easy to clean and doesn't absorb flavors and smells from ground items nor stain easily. If using the mortar and pestle for both magical and culinary mixtures, avoid grinding any toxic or inedible items in it, out of an abundance of caution.

To best use a mortar & pestle, place a small amount of the items you want to grind in the mortar. If you are grinding larger items, use kitchen shears to cut harder items into small pieces or a knife to chop softer items. For harder items like seeds, start by moving the pestle close to the seeds and lightly pound them until they have cracked. Make sure to keep the pestle close to the seeds while pounding, and don't use too much force or they will fly out of the mortar. Once the seeds are cracked, rotate the pestle around the mortar while pressing it in, until the mixture has been ground to the desired level.

Cleaning a stone mortar & pestle is relatively simple, but often uses a bit of elbow grease. Rinse both the pestle and mortar after use and allow to dry. Add a few tablespoons of uncooked white rice and grind. As the rice grinds, it will dislodge and absorb the remaining material in the mortar, turning a darker color. Discard the rice and add a few more tablespoons, and grind again. Once the ground white rice remains white, rinse the mortar and pestle and dry completely before storing.

Different Herbal Preparations Used in Wicca

Herbs are used in a multitude of different ways—depending on the spell used or needs of the practitioner. This section will describe several of these different preparations and include instructions on how to prepare herbs that way. Additionally, it will provide examples of how herbs are prepared and the different ways they can be used. Many of these methods are also used for culinary purposes, so feel free to use them to add an herbal punch to your next dinner.

Drying Herbs
A practitioner can use dried herbs in many ways. Among the most common are burning—as part of an incense during rituals or spells. This is best done using an incense charcoal with a comparable incense burner that can be purchased in some natural food stores as well as online. Pour a small amount of coarsely ground herbs on a charcoal tab in the incense burner and light the tab. Be cautious of overfilling the tab, it takes practice to learn the correct amount to use.

To air dry fresh herbs, harvest 6-10 branches of the herb and shake them out to remove any insects or soil. Bundle them together and tie the cut end tightly or use a rubber band. Place them in a paper bag, cut side up, and tie the bag closed. Puncture the bag in several places to provide airflow then hang the bag in a warm, well-ventilated area. Most herbs will dry in one to two weeks. You can also oven dry, though that cooks the herbs a bit—removing some of their essential oils.

Water-Based Herbal Mixtures

Combining herbs with water creates a mixture that the practitioner can use to provide an herbal punch to a variety of rituals and spells. For healing spells, mixtures can be applied to the skin over the area that needs healing, by soaking a cloth wrap in the herbal mixture and then wrapping the soaked cloth around the area. They can be added to bathwater or used to anoint tools and candles used in rituals. There are two basic types of water-based herbal mixtures: infusions and decoctions.

An ***infusion*** is the easier mixture to make. Simply combine dried herbs with water and allow it to sit. A general ratio of one tablespoon per cup of water works for most herbs, though some might need more or less to make a better infusion. This is something the practitioner will need to discover on their own, through practice. The amount of time the herbs are left in the water depends on the type of plant material. Harder plant matter like roots and bark often need about 8 hours, while leaves need about four. Flowers tend to require only 2 hours, while seeds and berries can create an infusion in under an hour. Once the time is up, strain the solids out of the infusion and store in a dark glass bottle.

A ***decoction*** takes a little more effort and

creates a more potent mixture. With a decoction, instead of leaving the plant matter in the water for a set amount of time, you will be boiling or simmering the mixture. This leaches more of the essential oils out of the plant matter, and with the loss of water through boiling, the mixture is further concentrated. To create an herbal decoction, use the same ration of herbs to water as the infusion, but put both into a saucepan and bring it to a boil. Once it boils, turn down the heat and allow it to simmer for anywhere from a half hour to two hours. Again, harder items need to be simmered longer, though simmering any material longer will help to make a stronger decoction.

An herbal infusion or decoction can be turned into an herbal simple syrup. The standard simple syrup is just an equal amount of water and sugar, heated until the sugar dissolves. Adding sugar to an herbal infusion or decoction can make drinking potent herbal mixtures much more palatable.

Oil-Based Herbal Mixtures

Herbal oils are used by practitioners in similar ways as a water-based infusion. They can be applied to the skin, used to anoint tools or even other people that are involved in certain rituals. The creation of herbal-infused oils requires a carrier or neutral oil. Olive oil has been used for this since ancient times, and it can be used now. Don't worry about using fancy extra virgin olive oil, unless you intend to consume your herb-infused oil. Grape seed and almond oil also make for good carrier oils.

For a simple ***cold infusion***, fill a clean canning jar half full with your desired herbs. Add your carrier oil until it covers the herbs. Seal the content tight and set in a sunny location. This can take up to a couple of weeks to infuse fully. Once that has been completed, strain the solids out of the oil and store in dark bottles, and store in a cool and dry place. Infused oils can last a year with proper storage.

A quicker method is a ***hot infusion***. The traditional method is to add the herbs and oil to the top of a double boiler and gently boil it for an hour. An easier method is in a slow cooker, set to warm. Prepare the herbs and oil in the same way as the cold infusion. Place a tea towel into your slow cooker and set the jars with the oil-herb mixtures on top of the towel. Fill the slow cooker with water until the water reaches just above the herb and oil mixture. Set the cooker on warm and leave for 8 to 10 hours. Let cool, strain and store in dark bottles, and store in a cool and dry place. Infused oils can last a year with proper storage.

These herbal infused oils can be made into a cream or lotion. This requires:

1 cup of herbal infused oil
4 ounces of bee's wax
.5 cup water
pinch of borax.

Heat the oil and bee's wax in a double boiler until the wax has fully melted. In another container, mix the borax and water together. Add a small amount of the water mixture into the double boiler and stir continuously. Keep adding a small amount of water until it has combined completely. Remove from heat and let cool. This lotion will likely be a bit oilier than commercially available lotions.

Alcohol-Based Herbal Mixtures

Herbal alcohol mixtures are not only incredibly useful for a practitioner of Wicca; they also form the base for most liqueurs. Chartreuse, the famous French liqueur, is an infusion of 130 different herbs and plants in distilled alcohol. Some alcohol-based herbal mixtures are meant to be drunk as part of a ritual or spell, but they can also be used for anointing tools or ritual participants.

Due to the volatility of alcohol when heated, a cold infusion is preferred, and like cold infused oil, it often takes a long time. With alcohol, it is called a tincture. Vodka is generally the spirit of choice in making a tincture, but rum is often used to add to the flavor. Using canning jars, fill the jar with herbs to about a third of the way, making sure they have been cut into small pieces to increase the amount of infusion. Pour a small amount of boiling water over the herbs and then fill the rest of the jar with the spirits. Store the jar in a cool dark place for at least 2 weeks. Make sure to shake the jars once a day. When finished, strain the solids and store in a dark glass bottle in a cool dark place for up to a year.

A tonic wine can be created in a similar manner. For each bottle of wine, add 6-8 oz. of fresh herbs. Store it for two weeks in a cool dark place before straining out the solids. Return the wine to a dark bottle and store in a cool and dark place.

If you're enjoying this book, I would appreciate it if you went to the place of purchase and left a short positive review. Thank you.

Chapter 3: Encyclopedia of Important Herbs Every Witch Should Understand

This chapter will contain a list of important magical plants with a short description of the plant, its magical qualities, and any caution against its use on the skin or internally. Most of the following herbs and plants are also common in food, but a few magical herbs are not recommended for internal use and that will be noted. People with medical conditions or on medications should be extra cautious and should perform a bit of research about the interactions between the herbs and their condition/medication before taking any internally.

Adder's Tongue
A relative of the lily, the adder's tongue is a fern-like plant with purple flowers and different species of it grow wild throughout the world. Known for its healing powers, it is often soaked in water and applied directly to bruises and included in other mixtures used for their healing properties.

Alfalfa
Known as Lucerne outside of North America, this perennial plant is commonly grown for animal feed and is a cousin to the clover. Its magical uses focus on prosperity. It is commonly used in

money spells, as well as other spells that are meant to bring prosperity. One simple method is to burn a small bunch of alfalfa and scatter the ashes in the wind at the four cardinal points of a property to bring those who live inside prosperity and wealth.

Allspice
A spice used extensively in Caribbean cooking, it is associated with luck as well as healing. It is often burnt as an incense to attract better luck or added to food as a healing agent.

Almond
The edible nut, as well as the leaves and branches, have magical properties that are often associated with wisdom and prosperity. Wands made of almond wood are common in some Wicca traditions.

Aloe
A flowering succulent, originally from the Arabian Peninsula. Its cultivation has spread throughout the world and it is a common houseplant. The gel harvested from inside its thick leaves is used extensively in skin creams as well as some food products. Magically, it is used for protection, often added to a wreath with other plants with protective powers and hung over or near the front door.

Anise
Native to the Mediterranean, Anise, with its licorice-like flavor, is commonly used to flavor

candy and liquor. Magically, it is associated with purification as well as protection. It is often added to purification baths as well as sleep sachets placed under the pillow at night to ward off bad dreams.

Apple
Apples play a major role in the fall festival of Samhain and, in Celtic mythology, represented immortality and considered the food of the dead. They are also commonly associated with love spells. Apple blossoms are commonly added to love sachets and can be used in incense. A simple apple love spell involves holding an apple in your hands until it has warmed and then giving the apple to the object of your infection. Apples are also associated with healing powers other than eating it; a slice of apple can be rubbed over injured areas to aid their healing.

Ash
It is an important tree in the mythology of Europe. Yggdrasil, the world tree in Norse mythology that connected all the different realms of the universe—was an ash tree. Ash is associated with healing and protection. Wands made of ash are commonly used in healing spells.

Avocado
The Avocado fruit is associated with lust and beauty. The ancient Aztecs considered it an aphrodisiac. Adding avocado oil into herbal skin creams will promote beauty, while the flesh can be added to mixtures intent on fuelling lust.

Balm, Lemon
It is a common ornamental plant that can be grown to attract bees. Its essential oil is commonly added to perfumes and candies. It is associated with love and healing. A tonic wine made with lemon balm and shared between friends is said to increase the strength of their bond. The dried lemon balm is often added to healing incenses.

Bamboo
Used extensively in Asia as a building material and as food, bamboo is a grass and is one of the fastest growing plants in the world. Associated with luck and protection, bamboo can be planted in gardens near homes to provide the residents good luck. It can be burned and scattered for protection and carving a personal symbol of luck on growing bamboo can grow your luck.

Barley
A common cereal grain used as food for both humans and livestock, it is one of the major ingredients used in the brewing of beer. Its magical uses focus on healing and protection. Barleycorns can be added to healing sachets or scattered around the outskirts of a property to protect the residents from negative energy.

Basil
An important culinary herb, it is the main ingredient in pesto and different varieties of basil are used in the foods of the Mediterranean as well as in Asia. Its magical associations are

equally broad, touching on love, protection, and prosperity. For love spells, basil can be added to perfumes, incenses, and sachets as part of spells to soothe disagreements between lovers. In medieval folklore, witches would drink basil juice before flying on their brooms.

Bay
The leaves of the bay plant are a common aromatic added to soups and stews for an extra burst of flavor. Magically, it is associated with prophecy and purification. Adding dry basil leaves to incense or sachets designed for purification will enhance their power. Prophetic dreams can be induced by adding dried bay leaves to a dream sachet placed under the pillow or hanging from the headboard.

Beans
An important and diverse crop of different legumes and one of the first crops ever cultivated by man, beans are also one of the three sisters along with corn and squash that formed the major crops grown by Native Americans. Associated with protection from malevolent spirits, Native Americans would construct rattles out of dried beans and rawhide. Sounding the rattle would ward off the evil spirits. Bean rattles can be made today for the same effect.

Beets
The roots are a common food in Eastern Europe and Central Asia, beets are known for their deep red color. Often associated with love spells,

beetroot juice can be used as ink in any love spell that requires writing. This juice can also be a safer substitute for blood in any spell that requires it.

Birch
A distinctive deciduous tree with its black-speckled, white bark, birch was the traditional wood used for witches' broom. Known for its powerful protection and purification qualities, birch twigs can be burned and the ashes can be spread around a property to protect the inhabitants. Shavings of the bark that are added to incense increase its powers of purification.

Blackberry
A common wild-growing, thorny vine with dark, raspberry-like, berries. Used for its powers of protection as well as for healing. Planting blackberry bushes near the home are thought to offer protection, but be careful, as they often grow like weeds and will take over a garden. Adding blackberry juice to healing tincture or infusions increases their potency.

Bluebell
A flowering plant named for its purplish blue, bell-shaped, flowers. It is closely associated with luck as well as protection. Bluebell flowers can increase one's luck by slipping one inside a shoe. Adding dried bluebell flowers to a sleep sachet will prevent nightmares.

Caraway
A member of the carrot family, its seed is often used to flavor a variety of different dishes in European and Middle Eastern cuisine. Magically, caraway seeds are used for their protective qualities as well as their connection with love. Adding caraway seeds to sachets can help to attract a mate. Growing caraway in a garden will ward the property from evil spirits.

Carrots
A common vegetable used worldwide in a variety of cuisines, carrot along with onion and celery form the mirepoix used as the base flavoring for classic French cuisine. Magically, it can be used to increase lust as well as fertility. Eating the seeds is a traditional way to encourage pregnancy in women.

Catnip
Named for its effect on felines, similar to a recreational drug, catnip has multiple magical properties including love, luck, and happiness. A common ingredient in love and friendship sachets, sharing it with your cat will increase the connection you both have. It can also be used as incense, although be cautious, as inhaling too much of the smoke can have a mild effect that is similar to when cats get a hold of some.

Cedar
A sacred tree to the Native Americans from the Pacific Northwest, it is known for its purifying and money related powers. Burning cedar

shavings provides a powerful purification smoke that can be used to rid rooms of negative energies. Carrying a small piece of cedar, often carved with personal symbols, in a purse or pocket will act as a draw for money.

Celery
A common vegetable used as the base flavoring of many cuisines, although magically, it promotes mental acuity and sound sleep. Celery seeds can be added to a sleep sachet. They can also be added to infusions or tinctures designed to increase concentration.

Chili peppers
The spicy cousin to the bell pepper, it used for its power to increase fidelity. Dried chili peppers can be added to sachets designed to return or reignite love.

Cinnamon
It is the edible bark of several different trees that provides a pungent kick to many different foods. Added to incense, it can offer a variety of magical aids including healing, protection, and luck. The essential oil is commonly used in several different cultures in religious ceremonies as anointing oil.

Clover
A common small flowering plant that is often associated with Ireland. Four-leaf clovers are traditionally considered lucky due to their rarity. Their magical powers include increasing success

and fidelity. Adding the dried leaves to sachets designed to increase success will enhance their power. A couple who consume a single clover together will find their love growing.

<u>Corn</u>
One of the most common grains grown today, corn was a staple from across the Americas and spread throughout the world after Columbus. Magically, it is used for its powers of protection. Dried ears of corn can be hung inside the house to protect its occupants. Corn pollen was tossed in the air to encourage rain by Native Americans in drier climates or during times of drought.

<u>Elder</u>
A flowering wild plant with dark red berries, Elder possesses many magical qualities and is useful for protection spells as well as those for better sleep and healing. Growing elder in the garden or hanging the branches in the home will ward off negative energies and spirits. The berries can be rubbed over areas of the body that ache and the leaves can be added to sleep sachets.

<u>Ferns</u>
Ferns are an interesting subset of plants that don't flower and grow wildly in most forests and jungles. Ferns are used by practitioners for their protective and purification powers. Dried ferns can be burned to purify an area. Planting ferns near the door to a home will offer protection from negative spirits.

Fig
The fig tree, a species of ficus is common throughout the world in warmer climates. Its fruit can be consumed fresh, but it is more commonly consumed dry. Magically, it is associated with love and fertility. A fig plant grown in the bedroom increases the love of those who sleep there, as well as their fertility.

Garlic
A cousin of the onion, its pungent bulbs are common to cuisine around the world. It possesses several magical qualities including protection, lust, and healing. Folklore holds that garlic protects against vampires, but this likely came from an earlier belief that garlic protected against the Black Death. Garlic can be used to ward against negative energies by placing it in the home, especially right after a move.

Ginger
A spicy root used in both savory and sweet dishes worldwide, ginger encourages success and wealth. Eating a small amount of raw ginger before casting a spell will add power to the cast, as well as increase the chances of success. Growing ginger in your garden can be an attractor of wealth.

Holly
This evergreen bush with thorny leaves is often associated with winter and Christmas because it remains green all year 'round. It is one of the more powerful protective herbs. Plant some holly

near the house to ward off negative energy. An infusion made from holly leaves can be sprinkled on people to protect them before they sleep. Hanging holly around the home in the winter is known to promote luck as well.

Hops
Hops are responsible for giving beer its slightly bitter bite. Their magical association is with promoting sleep. Dried hops are great additions to sleep sachets and sleep incenses.

Lavender
A small shrub with distinctive purple flowers, Lavender is used for its pleasant smell in perfumes, body products, and foods. Magically, it is associated with love, purification, and protection. Adding lavender to a love sachet or incense will increase its power. Rub fresh lavender flowers between your hands before a love ritual to increase its power and chances of success similarly. Dried lavender in incense acts as a purifier.

Lemon
The small tart yellow fruit of the lemon tree is a common citrus ingredient in cuisine worldwide. Making a water infusion by adding the juice and zest of a lemon to the water, it will become a powerful purifying agent that can be used to ritually purify tools and anoint people before performing a ritual or spell. Dried flowers and zest can add a citrus punch to sleep sachets of burned in incense.

Mandrake

Mandrake is the root of the Mandragora plant, common to the Mediterranean. The root of a mandrake bears a slight resemblance to a human. It contains an unpleasant hallucinogen that can cause an elevated heart rate and vomiting. For magical purposes, a whole mandrake root can be placed in a prominent area in the home, traditionally over the mantle or entrance to provide protection. Money placed near the mandrake root, especially silver coins, draws wealth to those who live in the home.

Mint

A family of herbs well known for their distinctive, crisp scent, its fresh taste is the reason why its used extensively in food. Magical mint is associated with wealth, healing, and protection. Fresh mint leaves can be kept in a wallet next to money to rub their scent and power into it. Mint leaves are also a common addition to healing concoctions. Mint oil can be used as anointing oil during healing rituals. Growing mint around the house offers protection, but do grow it in a pot—unless you want it to take over your garden!

Oak

A sacred tree in many different ancient cultures, the oak's acorns also provided many ancient people with a large and easily storable food source. Its magical attributes include protection, wealth, and healing. A wand made of oak provides more potency for protection spells. Both branches and acorns can be used in protective talismans. Planting an acorn during the full moon is part of a common spell designed to bring wealth.

Onion

One of the most ubiquitous vegetables in the world, the onion comes with a variety of magical attributes as well including protection, purification, and healing. Onions can be used to purify an Athame, simply rub a cut onion along the blade of the dagger. Similarly, rubbing the cut section of an onion over a bruise or pulled muscle will help heal it faster. Onion flowers can be added to protective incense and sachets.

Pine

A common evergreen tree often used as Christmas trees, pine can be used for its protection, purification, and healing powers. Pine needles can be burned as part of an incense to purify ritual spaces or homes. The needles can be added to healing baths or placed in a sleep sachet to grant protection from nightmares.

Rose

A flower often associated with romance and love, the rose's magical attributes also include healing and protection. Rose petals can be used in healing teas and water infusions can be mixed with other ingredients to make protective tonics. Dried rose petals make a wonderful addition to sleep sachets to heat up the libido in the bedroom.

Rosemary
Sacred to many ancient Mediterranean cultures, rosemary is used extensively in their cuisines today, as well as in fragrances. Magically, it possesses powers in protection, purification, love, and healing. Rosemary nettles added to sleep sachets protect the sleeper from nightmares and provide a healing sleep. It can be burned for its purification powers. Added to a bath, it provides both healing and protection. Washing the hands with rosemary infused water before performing healing spells are known to boost their power.

Sage
One of the four major herbs in British cuisine, sage is used throughout Europe and the Middle East in their foods. Magically, sage is known for its healing and purification qualities. Many Native American groups use a variety of sage for their smudge sticks and purifying incense. Burning ground sage leaves as part of a purification incense is also common. Sage infusions and tea can be taken for their healing effects.

Chapter 4: An Herbal Book of Shadows

In the modern Wiccan tradition, a witch's book of spells or **grimoire**—is known as their Book of Shadows. This chapter presents several spells that can be cast using herbs, so we can call it is our Herbal Book of Shadows. The following spells will be organized by type, with a section on love spells, wealth & luck spells, protection & healing spells, and sleep & dream spells.

Each spell will be presented in a similar fashion as a recipe book, with the necessary equipment listed before providing the steps to perform the spell. Spells can be performed as part of a greater ritual or with a more impromptu ritual. If casting a spell as part of an impromptu ritual, it is important to remember to include a purification aspect as well as casting the circle. Starting with a clean environment and clean tools will help ensure that no negative energies are attached before the spell is cast. Casting the circle protects the ritual space and its inhabitants from negative energy and spirits that magic sometimes attracts. Performing spells without these steps are just asking for the effect of your spells to be corrupted.

Another important aspect to understand is how magic works in the real world. This isn't fantasy magic where you can cast a spell to break the laws of physics or that will enslave someone's mind and making them love you. Think of real magic as a way to increase the odds. Casting a spell to attract money, for example, will make the odds of money finding you more in your favor.

You also get more from your magical endeavors when you put more effort to bring about the desired effect without magic as well. Take the wealth spell from the last paragraph, for example. If you cast this spell and then go sit on the couch, doing nothing, just expecting and waiting for it to bring wealth into your life—then the spell will likely fail because you have not provided an avenue for wealth to find you. There are also situations like this where, when the spell has no other avenue to work with, it will create one. Maybe a great aunt will pass away leaving some money for you. That is generally not how you would want wealth to find you.

Herbal Love Spells

Spells designed to bring love into one's life and to strengthen the existing bonds of love and friendships are among the most popular spells in Wicca. Remember to put in the effort and not just rely on magic to improve your love life. Magic is a tool that you can use to enhance, not a guarantee.

Honey Jar Attraction Spell

This is a spell designed to attract the interest of a specific person, although, with a slight modification, it can be used to attract the love of an unknown person.

Items required:

- Honey
- A Jar with a tight-fitting lid
- Love related herbs and flowers (rose petals and basil for example)
- Paints and supplies used to decorate the jar
- A Pen
- A Small slip of paper
- A pink candle

Instructions:

1. Begin by cleaning and purifying the jar.

Using cleansing incense and then salted water will work here though if you have a cleansing method you prefer, that is perfectly acceptable.
2. Decorate the jar with symbols or representations of love. These tend to be personal but can also use standard love symbols like red or pink hearts.
3. Write the name of the person you want to attract on the slip of paper and place it inside the jar. If you want to attract the love of a new person, write a few words describing the type of person whose love you want on the slip of paper.
4. Place the paper in the jar and add the herbs and petals.
5. Pour honey into the jar and seal it. You don't need to fill the whole jar with honey, just enough to coat the herbs and slip of paper.
6. If you are seeking the love of a specific person, carve their initials into the pink candle.
7. Take the jar and place it on your altar, placing the pink candle on top of it.
8. Cast a circle and light the candle.
9. Let the candle burn out and move the jar to your bedroom, placing it in a prominent place.
10. Recharge the spell every couple of weeks by returning the jar to the altar and burning another pink candle on top of it.

Herbal Love Perfume

This is a perfume meant to attract love and is best created about a week before the full moon. Different herbs can be used if you prefer a different scent, but sticking with herbs that are associated with love will help keep the perfume potent. The choice of alcohol can be changed as well.

Items Required:

- A small glass jar with a tight lid
- Brandy
- Cheesecloth or strainer
- Cloves
- Cardamom seeds
- Rose petals
- A cinnamon stick
- Dark glass bottle, with a dropper
- A red cloth

Instructions:

1. Lightly pulverize the cinnamon stick with a mortar and pestle before adding the other herbs. Give them a few rotations, just to break them up a little.
2. Pour the herbs onto the red cloth and add the rose petals.
3. Place the cloth on top of the altar.
4. Cast your circle and hold your hands on

top of the herb and cloth.
5. Envision the love you have and want to share, gather the energy into your hands, and push it into the herbs.
6. Unwrap the herbs and place them into the small jar.
7. Fill the jar with brandy and put the lid on tight.
8. Move the jar to a cool dark place in your bedroom, if possible, and shake it once a day.
9. Open the jar on the day of the full moon.
10. Strain the solids out of the perfume and store it in a dark glass bottle with a dropper.
11. To attract love, wear a drop of perfume on each wrist and wherever else you would normally wear perfume.

Spell for Burning Desire

This is a spell designed to reignite the love and passion between an established couple.

Items Required:

- Vanilla extract
- A red candle
- Cloves
- A hot chili pepper, fresh

Instructions:

1. Carve both your initials as well as your lover's into the candle with your Athame—careful to avoid cutting yourself. Your blood and pain from such an accident are counterproductive for the spell.
2. Place a drop of vanilla extract on your finger and rub it against the candle to anoint it.
3. Press several cloves into the top half of the candle.
4. Cut the pepper in half and rub the cut side against the bottom half of the candle. If you do not regularly use hot peppers, donning gloves when handling them might be advisable, otherwise, make sure to wash your hands thoroughly afterward and do not rub your eyes or nose before.
5. Take the candle to your altar and cast a circle.

6. Light the candle and stare into the flame for a moment, envisioning the heat of the candle's flame feeding the passion you and your partner feel for each other.
7. Once you have finished your envisioning, blow out the candle.
8. Move the candle to your bedroom and light again before getting amorous with your partner.

Herbal Wealth & Luck Spells

Spells designed to attract wealth are almost as popular as love spells. Remember the warning above about working with the spells. Don't just cast a spell to attract wealth, and then do nothing to bring about wealth. Luck and wealth often go hand in hand, so this section also includes a couple of luck spells. These can be used to increase your luck in a variety of ways, not just for financial gain.

Chalice of Plenty

This is a good wealth-attracting spell to perform if you have a garden, as the contents of the chalice need to be poured out onto a growing plant. This will have the added benefit of transferring some of the residual power into the growing plant. The wealth attracting energies imbued in the plant will make it a powerful plant to use in wealth spells as it grows. The milk used in this spell can be replaced with soy or nut milk, should you not desire to use animal milk.

Items Required:

- Milk
- A sprig taken from an oak tree
- A small smooth river or sea stone
- A wine glass or silver chalice

Instructions:

1. Clean and purify the goblet, oak sprig, and stone.
2. Cast the circle and place the goblet on the altar.
3. Fill the goblet with milk.
4. Hold the small stone above the goblet and envision golden energy coming from your hand, entering the stone. See this energy as a magnet for wealth and prosperity.
5. Once you have filled the stone with energy, gingerly drop it into the chalice.
6. Take the sprig of oak and swirl the milk with it three times, envisioning the golden light from the stone moving into the milk.
7. Let the chalice sit on the altar for a day and then pour it over a growing plant in your garden.

Money Sachet Spell

This spell creates a sachet, which is a small cloth bag filled with herbs. Sachets are commonly placed near something that represents the intent of the spell. For wealth spells the best place to put the sachet is near your wallet, so in your purse or wallet.

Items Required:

- 3 silver coins
- A green candle
- 7 basil leaves
- 7 allspice berries
- A pinch of ground cinnamon
- A pinch of ground ginger
- A small green cloth bag

Instructions:

1. Cast your circle and place all of the ingredients on the altar.
2. Light the green candle and envision your wealth growing.
3. Drop the three coins into the bag followed by the rest of the ingredients.
4. Hold the bag to your chest and stare into the candle flame, continuing to envision your wealth growing.
5. Blow out the candle and keep the sachet near your wallet.
6. Repower the sachet by returning the

candle to the altar and envisioning wealth energy returning to the sachet.

The Money Orange

This spell uses a penny and it is important to the spell that the penny is given away at the end. A store with a take a penny/leave a penny tray works for this, as well as just dropping it somewhere it is likely to be found. If possible, perform this spell using a found penny. This enhances the powers of luck involved.

Items Required:

- An orange
- A brown candle
- Cinnamon
- Basil
- A penny
- A slip of paper

Instructions:

1. Cast your circle and envision a golden aura surrounding you, bringing with it luck and wealth.
2. Write one or two of the things you would do with more money on the slip of paper.
3. Place the penny on the paper and sprinkle the basil and cinnamon over it.
4. Fold the paper over the penny and continue to fold it over the penny until it is cocooned in the paper.
5. Carefully make a slit in the orange with your Athame and slide the cocooned

penny inside the orange.
6. Hold the orange to your chest and envision the golden aura again, this time push it into the orange.
7. Close the circle and place the orange in a prominent place that you associate with money. Maybe near where you leave your wallet at home
8. After 7 days take the coin out and give it away.

Luck Pouch

This is another sachet spell but the resulting pouch is tied to a growing tree. The luck created with the spell will grow as the tree does.

Items Required:

- An Acorn
- A river stone
- A slip of paper
- Pen with Green ink
- A small green cloth bag
- A coin

Instructions:

1. Place the paper on the altar and draw a pentagram on it with green ink.
2. Write your name around the border of the pentagram and place the coin on top.
3. Fold the paper around the coin and place it in the bag.
4. Draw a pentagram on the acorn and place it along with the stone into the bag.
5. Close the bag and hold it to your chest envisioning the energies of luck entering the bag and charging the items.
6. When they are sufficiently charged, tie the bag around the branch of a growing tree.

Good Luck Bath

This bath will provide luck for at least the day after taking it. Perform the luck bath before a big job interview or meeting at work for it to go your way.

Items Required:

- A large pot or saucepan
- A teapot full of boiling water
- A strainer
- Nutmeg
- Cloves
- 1-inch chunk of Ginger root
- A Cinnamon stick

Instructions:

1. Coarsely ground the cinnamon stick, ginger root, and cloves with a mortar & pestle, adding ground nutmeg at the end.
2. Place all of the ingredients on the altar.
3. Envision a golden aura surrounding you and move that aura to the items in the mortar & pestle.
4. Pour the contents of the mortar into a pot then add the boiling water.
5. Let this steep for at least an hour then draw a bath.
6. Pour the infusion into the water, through a strainer to remove any solids.
7. Enter the bath and soak until it cools

slightly, continuing to envision the success and luck you will have in your endeavors that day or the next.

Herbal Protection & Health Spells

The following spells fall into two categories: Protection spells that ward the home against negative energy, or actively attract positive energy and healing spells designed to aid the body's healing powers.

Home Protection Spell

This is a spell to perform when you first move into a new home or when the energies inside the home just do not feel right. Dried herbs work best in this spell, and you only need a small amount of each.

Items Required:

- Sea Salt
- Lavender
- Rosemary
- Basil
- 4 small bowls to hold the herbs
- A White Candle

Instructions:

1. Take all of the ingredients and place them on your altar.
2. Cast the circle and light the white candle.

3. Let it burn for a few minutes while envisioning a shimmering shield forming over your home.
4. Blow out the candle and leave the herbs on the altar until sunrise.
5. At sunrise, take the bowl with the sea salt to the north side of your property and sprinkle the salt.
6. Move to the west side of your property with the lavender and sprinkle it.
7. Now, move to the south with the rosemary, sprinkling it at the southern edge of your property.
8. Finally, move to the east side of the property with the basil, and sprinkle it at the edge.

Witch Jar

This is an old spell designed to protect the residents of a property from both negative energies, as well as malevolent spellcasters. The negative energies are drawn to the bottle where the rusty nails and shards of glass trap them allowing the rosemary to banish them.

Items Required:

- A small jar with a tight-fitting lid
- Soured wine
- Rusty nails
- Broken glass
- Rosemary
- A brown candle

Instructions:

1. Soak the jar in salted water to purify it.
2. Fill the jar with the rusty nails and broken glass.
3. Take the jar to your altar and cast the circle.
4. Light the brown candle.
5. Sprinkle the rosemary into the jar while envisioning the negative energies and evil spirits to be trapped.
6. Pour the soured wine into the bottle and seal it tightly.
7. Move the brown candle to the top of the bottle and let it burn out.

8. Retrieve the bottle from your altar and bury it near the front door to your home.

Positivity Magnet Spell

This spell is designed to attract positive energy. This can be a boost for luck as well as general health.

Items Required:

- 1 silver candle
- A small fireproof bowl
- Magnet
- Slip of paper
- Pen
- Pine needles

Instructions:

1. Take all of the ingredients to your altar and cast the circle.
2. Light the candle and envision positive energy growing inside yourself.
3. Write a desire on the slip of paper, one that more positive energy would help bring about.
4. Set the magnet on the slip of paper with your desire written on it and sprinkle the pine needles over it.
5. Wrap the magnet in the paper and continue to envision positive energy growing and now moving into the paper-wrapped magnet.
6. Unwrap the paper and set the magnet aside.

7. Place the paper into the fire-proof bowl with the pine needles still on top of it.
8. Carefully light the paper with the silver candle.
9. Carry the magnet close to you for the next week to attract positive energies.

Healing Power of Three Spell

This speed can be used to aid in the healing of others or yourself. The colors of the candles used can differ based on the illness or ailment. The final chapter has further resources where you can learn more about which colors are associated with different ailments.

Items Required:

- Mint Oil
- Sandalwood Oil
- Myrrh Oil
- A slip of paper
- Pen or pencil
- Three candles in healing colors.

Instructions:

1. Take all the ingredients to your altar and cast the circle.
2. Set the candles up in a triangle on your altar.
3. Anoint each candle with one of the essential oils; this only needs a drop or two of each.
4. Write the name of the person who needs healing on the slip of paper and place it in the center of the altar.
5. Light the three candles and envision the healing powers of the spell, healing their ailment, returning them to good health.

6. Let the candles burn for three hours before blowing them out.

Beauty Bath

This bath can be used to improve your confidence and make you feel as beautiful as you can be. In any bath that uses herbs, it is a good idea to have a tub strainer in the drain of your tub to catch any leaves. This will also prevent hair clogs for added benefits.

Items Required:

- .5 cup marigold petals
- .5 cups raspberry leaves
- A teacup
- Three yellow Candles
- A kettle with boiling water

Instructions:

1. Take the petals and leaves to your altar and cast the circle.
2. Envision power entering the leaves and petals, boosting your confidence and beauty.
3. Draw a bath and set the three yellow candles around the bathtub or as close, yet as safely possible.
4. Add half of the petals and leaves to the bath water.
5. Put the other half into the teacup and pour the boiling water into the cup.
6. Enjoy your bath and drink your tea, continuing to envision the energies in the leaves and petals melting into your body

Herbal Dream and Sleep Spells

The following spells produce sachets that can be kept under your pillow to increase the quality of your sleep or to induce dreams. If you are a fidgety sleeper and move a lot in your sleep, having the sachets on your headboard will likely serve you better. If a sachet bursts under your pillow, spreading its herbal contents all over your bed, it will not do much to improve your sleep.

Herbal Dream Sachet

Items Required

- A small purple cloth pouch
- Chamomile
- Lavender
- Hops
- Cloves
- Jasmine
- Dried rose petals

Instructions:

1. Take all of the ingredients to your altar and cast the circle.
2. Place all of the ingredients into the purple cloth pouch and set it on the altar
3. Set your hands over the cloth pouch and envision the pouch granting you happy and restful dreams, with no nightmares if

you are plagued by them.
4. Set it under your pillow or hanging from your headboard for happier dreams.
5. Recharge it on your altar when it loses its effect.

Herbal Sleeping Sachet Spell

Similar to the dream sachet, this one is more for restful sleep than inducing dreams.

Items Required:

- A small purple cloth pouch
- 7 cloves
- .5 oz. rosemary
- 7 cardamom pods
- Pinch of sea salt
- A pink candle
- A purple candle
- A white candle

Instructions:

1) Place the candles in a triangle on your altar with the other ingredients inside the triangle.
2) Cast your circle and light the candles, envisioning a restful sleep.
3) Pour the ingredients into the bag while continuing to envision a restful and recharging sleep.
4) Blow out the candle and place the sachet under your pillow or hanging from your headboard.
5) Recharge at your altar when it loses its effect.

If you're enjoying this book, I would appreciate it if you went to the place of purchase and left a short positive review. Thank you.

Chapter 5: Where to Buy and How to Grow & Forage Herbs for Magical Usage

For the sourcing of herbs, the modern magical practitioner has a multitude of choices that are almost completely unavailable to the practitioners of even the recent past. Spices and herbs from halfway across the world are processed and shipped in a fraction of time compared to the older methods. For example, a round trip from Italy to China on the Silk Road took about 2 years to complete. Now, cargo ships can make the same round trip in less than two weeks and a round-trip flight clocks in at just less than 20 hours.

In addition to just buying herbs and other plants, the modern practitioner has many more options when it comes to growing them. Seeds from all over the world are easily obtainable, and with the lowering costs for grow lamps, growing herbs inside—that require a warmer climate than the practitioner's garden provides—is an affordable option.

Finally, the modern practitioner can gather their herbs from their surroundings, foraging like the practitioners of olden times. Even here, there are benefits for the modern practitioner. There are books detailing the different medicinal and magical herbs that can be found in each region of the United States as well as the rest of the world. With one of these guides in hand, the practitioner can source some of their herbs from their environment.

This chapter will look into all three ways the modern practitioner of magic can source their herbs and other plants. It will provide tips for each of the three ways, as well as delving into the pros and cons, along with any safety warnings when needed.

Buying Herbs

The simplest option for gathering herbs a practitioner needs for their spell work is buying them. Herbs can be purchased from a variety of different sources: grocery stores, herbalists, ethnic markets, spice shops, natural food stores, and of course, the internet. All of these offer herbs of differing quality and equally differing costs. Some practitioners find herbs of lower quality, which negatively affect their spells, while others put less stock into the quality of the herbs, the best way to determine the quality of herbs required for your spells takes experimentation.

Most modestly stocked grocery stores offer a variety of dried herbs and spices as well as a modest amount of the most commonly used fresh culinary herbs. Many include a small floral section where flower petals and leaves can be purchased as part of bouquets. As most people live close enough to one of these grocery stores, availability is a real pro. Unfortunately, the cost of dried herbs and spices at these stores tends to be exorbitantly high and you have little ability to buy specific amounts. Most of their herbs and spices are sold in small bottles instead of loose. Fresh herbs often fall into the same problem with the stores selling small containers of most of the fresh herbs.

Ethnic grocery stores often provide a better option for buying dried herbs and spices. These stores cater to the cuisine and other products of people who come from a specific region and are more likely to provide a greater variety than standard groceries, and their herbs and spices are often less expensive and available for bulk purchasing, enabling the consumer to buy only the amount they need instead of a bottle. Three of the most common ethnic stores in the Unified States are Latin American, Indian, and Asian. Most Latin American and Asian markets offer products used throughout the region instead of specifying a single country; in larger cities, more specialized stores are not uncommon. Asian markets usually offer foods and goods from the major countries in East Asia, including China, South Korea, Japan, the Philippines, Vietnam, and Thailand, though some offer goods from other countries as well.

The spices in ethnic stores will sometimes be much fresher than those in standard groceries. These stores often source their herbs and spices directly from international producers that ship their products directly from the processing plant.

The biggest downside to ethnic stores is that the herbs and spices available will generally be limited to those used in the cuisine of the area. Another downside to ethnic groceries is finding them. They are prevalent in large cities, but only common in smaller towns that have a large enough population of the specific ethnicity to support the store.

Buying herbs and spices from dedicated spice stores offers the greatest variety of choices as well as some of the highest quality of herbs and spices, depending on the store. Most spice shops offer the option to purchase the spices whole or ground. From a culinary aspect, once the spice is ground, the oils inside are exposed to air and it starts to lose its flavor potency slowly. Some feel the same about the magical qualities, for example, purchasing whole spices to be ground later as part of an infusion used in a spell will provide more power to the spell than purchasing the same spices ground.

Most spice shops offer their goods in bulk allowing the consumer to purchase only the amount they need. The prices can often be daunting, spices in spice shops can often go for $30-$50 a pound and higher, but most spells only require a fraction of that amount. The biggest downside to spice shops is their availability. Most large cities have one or two dedicated spice shops, but they are rare outside those big cities. Thankfully, most of the better ones sell online, so those who live in a more rural area still have access. Another con is that spice shops only sell culinary herbs and spices, so they make poor choices for those hunting for nonculinary herbs.

One of the best options for buying magical herbs and plants is a store that specializes in magical or occult products. Like spice stores, these tend to be found in major metropolises and can sometimes be difficult to find as they go by many different names such as herbalists, occult bookstores, metaphysical stores... These stores often have a large selection of herbs for use in magic, as well as having salespersons that are familiar with the magical practice who can offer tips and suggestions. They also carry a large variety of books and magical tools to continue your metaphysical education. Their prices tend to be more expensive than spice shops and ethnic grocers, but less expensive than standard grocery stores. If you have access to one, it will likely become your go-to place for buying herbs.

Growing Herbs

Growing your own herbs takes a bit more time than purchasing, but you are in control of their quality, and adding your own hard work to grow the herbs you use in your spells, add a personal element that can contribute to the power of the spells. In addition, most gardens produce more herbs than you will need in your spells, allowing you to eat the rest, adding a culinary benefit, too.

Before planting anything in your garden, it is

helpful to determine your area's plant hardiness zone. For the United States, the USDA provides an interactive online map to determine this, and the link is included in the resources in the next chapter. The plant hardiness zone will determine what you can plant in that climate and when you should plant. Seed packets usually include what zones they can grow in so you can use that to better plan your garden.

Many herbs make great houseplants and can be grown in a sunny spot of the home. LED grow lights have been decreasing in costs with small ones that include a timer available for under $30. These inexpensive lamps allow for the growing of herbs that need more light or higher temperatures than what is available in your climate. Some more traditional practitioners feel that the use of grow lamps hampers the magical powers of the herbs since the sun isn't involved. If you find yourself in that camp, limit your grow light use for culinary herbs.

Foraging for Herbs

The final way to procure herbs is to forage for them in your local environment. On the positive side, the cost of this is just your time and hunting for specific wild plants can be both good exercise and a calming activity. On the other hand, the selection will be limited to the plants native to your area. Additionally, some plants are poisonous to humans, so foraging for wild plants that will be consumed can be dangerous to those who do not know their local plants.

For those interested in foraging for their own plants, the next chapter provides several books specific to the plants of different regions of the United States. Picking up a copy of one of these books for your area will allow you to find the correct plants better. There are often groups or classes in wild plants available locally. Joining one of those groups or taking those classes will better prepare you for foraging for your own herbs.

Chapter 6: Further Resources

For those looking for further resources about Wicca—in general, herbs and plants in Wicca, and foraging wild plants, the following books are wonderful places to get more specialized knowledge.

Books on Wicca and Magic:

Witchcraft Today by Gerald Gardner

Gerald Gardner was one of the founders of the modern Wicca tradition, and *Witchcraft Today* provides a wonderful foundation for those looking to tread further down the path of Wicca.

Wicca: A Guide for the Solitary Practitioner by Scott Cunningham

An introduction to Wicca and its practices, intended for those who want to explore it alone instead of in a coven or other group of practitioners. The author's *Book of Shadows* is included as well.

Buckland's Complete Book of Witchcraft by Raymond Buckland

A more advanced book on practical Wicca, it

contains extensive instruction on a variety of different types of spellwork as well as the history and lore of Wicca.

Cunningham's Encyclopedia of Magical Herbs by Scott Cunningham

Another classic by the late Scott Cunningham, one of modern Wicca's most prolific authors in his short life, this is the ultimate guide to over 400 magical plants and herbs including how they can be used in spells and other magical ways.

Condensed Chaos: An Introduction to Chaos Magic by Phil Hine

For those more interested in a more improvisatory magical tradition, *Chaos Magic* might be for you and *Condensed Chaos* is the best source to start learning about this more anarchic tradition of magic.

Books on Foraging for Plants:

The wild plants available for foraging depend heavily on the area where you are foraging. Below are some books with region-specific information for the United States. International readers will likely find similar books for their country/region widely available.

- ***Field Guide to Edible Wild Plants by Bradford Angier***

- ***Medicinal Plants of the Western Mountain States by Charles W. Kane***

- ***Wild Edible Plants of Texas: A Pocket Guide to the Identification, Collection, Preparation, and Use of 60 Wild Plants of the Lone Star State by Charles W. Kane***

- ***Medicinal Plants of the American Southwest (Herbal Medicine of the American Southwest) by Charles W. Kane***

- ***Southern California Food Plants: Wild Edibles of the Valleys, Foothills, Coast, and Beyond by Charles W. Kane***

- ***Pacific Northwest Foraging: 120 Wild and Flavorful Edibles from Alaska Blueberries to Wild Hazelnuts by Douglas Deur***

- ***Pacific Northwest Medicinal Plants: Identify, Harvest, and Use 120 Wild Herbs for Health and Wellness by Scott Kloos***

- ***Midwest Foraging: 115 Wild and Flavorful Edibles from Burdock to Wild Peach (Regional Foraging Series) by Lisa M. Rose***

- ***Northeast Foraging: 120 Wild and Flavorful Edibles from Beach Plums to Wineberries (Regional Foraging Series) by Leda Meredith***

- ***Southeast Foraging: 120 Wild and Flavorful Edibles from Angelica to Wild Plums (Regional Foraging Series) by Chris Bennett***

Resources for Growing Plants

Before planting new herbs, vegetables or other plants in your garden, checking on your area's plant hardiness zone help to determine what plants will thrive in your area, as well as the best time of the year to plant them. For the United States, the United States Department of Agriculture provides an interactive online map you can use to find what zone you live in.

For international readers, your government might provide similar information to allow you to learn what and when to plant your garden.

Conclusion

Thank you for making it through to the end of *Herbal Magic: Wicca Beginner guide to Herbs and plants for Rituals and Spells*, I hope you found it informative as an introduction to the use of herbs and other plants in Wiccan magical practice.

This book barely scratched the surface of the information available on Wicca, so if you are interested in further study, the sky is the limit. Looking for Wiccan groups near you to join, or even just to ask for more information is a great place to continue your study of Wicca, and of course, the books listed in the last chapter are great ways to learn more.

www.ingramcontent.com/pod-product-compliance
Lightning Source LLC
Chambersburg PA
CBHW020545080526
44583CB00013B/996